Gourmet
ALKALINE

William Wallace

BALBOA.
PRESS

A DIVISION OF HAY HOUSE

Balboa Press books may be ordered through booksellers or by contacting:

Balboa Press
A Division of Hay House
1663 Liberty Drive
Bloomington, IN 47403
www.balboapress.com
1 (877) 407-4847

ISBN: 978-1-9822-2688-6 (sc)
ISBN: 978-1-9822-2689-3 (e)

Print information available on the last page.

Balboa Press rev. date: 05/01/2019

Dedication

To those who understand the importance of 9 Star Ki, the teachings and books of Michio Kushi, Dr. Hulda Clark, Hanna Kroeger and everyone who believes in natural healing, is for PH food labeling, who buys this book and let people live and let live.

And especially to the Magnet Magnificent
Glenn Marshall Wood
"Thanks for Everything"

Disclaimer

This publication does not condone the violation of any legitimate laws of these united States of America. This book is published under the 1st Amendment of the Constitution. I am not a licensed doctor of any kind. All materials in this book are written in great faith with no intent to mistreat anyone. Do not believe anything anyone tells you until you have checked it out yourself. When trying to solve a problem, look for the largest common denominator. In my investigation all the problems are with acidic PH people. They are unbalanced mentally and physically. All the prosperous people are alkaline. Especially if your PH was at least 8. At any rate proof is in the high alkaline pudding.

Digestion

Almost everyone is overweight because of improper digestion. It's not what you eat but how you eat it. There are 10 types of digestive enzymes.

- Seafood
- Beef, pork, deer, bison
- Elk, fowl, pepper
- Lamb, goat, salt
- Eggs, nuts, almond and cashew milk
- Rice, oats, flour, millet, wheat, quinoa, garlic, soy
- Beans, legumes, chickpeas, green peas
- Vegetables and fruits
- Sugar, drugs
- Dairy

Apples and peaches are neutral.

Each meal should not be more than 4 digestive enzymes up to age 45, then 3 after age 45. More than that will put extra labor on the heart. It must be more than ½ an ounce to count. After 50 times changing the digestive enzymes back and forth, the body will give up on digestion or have a heart attack. What doesn't get digested turns to fat. Drink before and after a meal. During dilutes digestive enzymes. If you need something to drink, sip water.

The birth of a child is determined by which parent is more yin. However to have a boy at month 8 for 36 days eat 6oz beef or bison, 2 eggs, and 4oz butter beans. It can be in 3 separate meals. If you have heartburn it means you didn't chew your food enough. Swallow some saliva. Eating your meals with family helps digestion by 20% from the family energy. A family that eats together stays together.

Brain

The brain changes 6 times. There is a big difference in age 18 to 21 which is why the founding fathers made the voting age 21. 50% of the male and female brains are the same. A third of the female brain is for raising children. Female brains are wired where all their experiences are connected which is great if they don't have any bad experiences. Males can departmentalize everything, concentrating on one thing at a time. 16 year old boys are responsible for 1 automobile death a week, 16 year girls 1 a day. Why? They have a harder time concentrating on one thing. Save lives by raising girls' driving age to 17. Their brains need an extra year of development. Watch YouTube – A Tale of Two Brains by Mark Gungor. If the draft age in the Vietnam War had remained 21 there would have 12,000 less casualties because of a more mature brain. If the politicians were alkaline there would have been zero casualties. Also the bankers and colleges could not take advantage of you. The average college grad owes $200,000. Thank you, Congress.

Growth of Brain

Age 4th month pregnancy to birth – 40%
Age 0-2 –25% (baby years)
Age 3-12 – 10% (the discipline years)
Age 13-19 – 10% (teen years)
Age 20 – 5% (pre adult year)

Age 21-25 – 10% (adult years)

50% of the male and female brain is the same.
20% at birth
10% the baby years
10% the child years
10% the teen years

5.6 PH

Anxiety – problems with kidneys and appendix
8 oz. watermelon/1 month with 2 milk thistles/1 month plus 10 days

If you have another baby in 13 months or less and the mother's PH is below 7.5 there is an 80% chance of post partem blues.

Most Creative Time with at least an 8 PH

Capricorn – 6-10 AM
Aquarius – 7-11 PM
Pisces – 7-11 AM
Aries – 3-7 PM
Taurus – 5-9 PM
Gemini – 3-7 PM
Cancer – 8PM-Midnight
Leo – 8PM-Midnight
Virgo – 5-9 AM
Libra – 6-10PM
Scorpio – Midnight-4AM
Sagittarius – 4-8PM
Both times if born on the cusp

School Program

With alkaline students, school lunches should be at least 8.5 PH.

You are capable of learning the most the first 5 years of your life. You're over the hill at 6.

Out of the 26 school systems, the USA is 23rd and #1 for amount spent on each student. This incompetence has been going on for over 60 years. It is like someone wants you to be raised stupid.

Schooling should start at age 5. The class should have 6 students with everyone the same sex and sign, including the teacher. This will reinforce who you are. At age 8 or 9 it will change to 12 students, all the same sex and sign including the teacher. At age 10 to 16 it will change to 24, with mixed sex and signs. Graduate at age 16. Age 17 take a year off, go to college or learn a trade than can put you through college.

Math ages 6, 7, 8, 13 and 16
English ages 6 to 10, 13 to 16
Music – start with violin – ages 6 to 16 (ask Santana)
Dance Boys and girls age 5 – 10, 1 hour 3 to 5 days a week
8-9 PH energy – Weight Lifting Boys and girls 16 – 17, 3 hours 2x/week
Chess ages 8 to 12

Foreign language ages 10 to 13

Sports ages 8 to 16, contact sports ages 14 to 16

Science ages 10 to 16

Home female economics ages 12 to 14

History ages 12 to 16

Puzzles ages 5, 8 to 12

Speech ages 5 to 6

Singing ages 5 to 8

Gardening ages 12 to 16

This program will reduce school cost by 30%, up their IQ by a minimum of 95 points, making the U.S. first in education and third in cost, and that's with free lunches. By keeping an alkaline PH of at least 8 prevents disease. Students need their summer off. School should not start until September. Every year their summer vacation gets shorter and shorter. They need their summer vacation mentally and physically. Why? They are still growing and are not adults yet.

If the government is going to let people at 18 with an underdeveloped brain vote, the higher the PH of the voter, the better off the country would be.

Age 14 is the age of 24/7 supervision.

Girls – 3 hours a week with horses, 3 hours a week dancing, sports, 5 hours a week art. Keep active.

Boys – military school. If breast fed, will make an extra $75,000/year at age 30, not breast fed $55,000/year. If you're an eagle scout, add $20,000/year whether breast fed or not. Eagle scouts very rarely get divorced, are balanced, and have a joyful life.

Private school students have a higher GPA because their diet is 30% more alkaline. This gives them a higher IQ making them an extra $30,000/year at age 30. This is for both sexes.

Hormone Changes

For the age of 13 and for the female change which should be at age 45 and last for 145 days.

Tomatoes – 4oz/day whole cooked carrots without 4oz/day squash 6oz/day will make change 1/3 easier.

Puberty is at age 13 years 6 month to 14 years 11 months. Listed hardest to easiest are Scorpio, Taurus, Leo, Pisces, Gemini, Sagittarius, Virgo, Aries, Libra, Cancer, Capricorn and Aquarius.

Below 6 PH

Abortions

30% do not know who the father is. 60% know but the father doesn't care. 20% think the baby will be born with birth defects where it is actually less than 1%. 80% feel abandoned. 30% regret having abortions and think it's wrong.

95% are scared. 80% are on drugs. 100% don't want the baby. They don't love themselves and are incapable of loving a baby. 85% of Americans think abortion is up to the person. 65% of Americans think it's morally wrong but it's not their body and none of their business. The American public should not have to pay for something that they think is morally wrong. Less than ½ of 1% of American women have abortions. Charles Manson's mother tried to get an abortion in 3 different states.

Government Employees

If joining the military, water signs should join the navy, earth signs join the army, air signs join the air force, and fire signs make great firemen or policemen. If born on the cusp of air and water, you should be an air craft carrier pilot. All pilots should have a PH of at least 8.5. This would reduce crashes by 70%, eliminating pilot error. Anyone operating a firearm should have a PH of at least 8.5. This would reduce deaths by 40%. Why? Balance people don't make mistakes.

Average Postal worker 6.5

Most Fireman 8.6

Most Policeman 6.8

Most Policewoman 6.3

Most Male politician 7.1

Most Female politician 6.3

Average female republican 8.9

Average male republican 8.5

Average female democrat 6.5

Average male democrat 6.9

Average Independent 9.1 PH

Average sovereign Citizen 8.9 PH

Average female flight pilot 7.9

Average male flight pilot 8.6

Most Prisoner guards 6.5

Most Astronauts 8.9

Average DFCS workers 5.3

Average Inmates 6.5

Average TSA 6.1

President Donald Trump 8.5 PH

Founding Fathers 8.9 – no processed food

7.8 PH

Johnson & Johnson Baby Powder

Alkaline doesn't cause cancer. There are hundreds of million people who have used the powder and did not get cancer. It is impossible for anything alkaline to cause cancer. Only acidic causes cancer at 5.4 PH and below. The powder is for external use but if digested it alkalizes the stomach and acts as an anti-acid.

7 dust 3.1 PH

Roundup - 5.7 PH

Sugar – 4.8 – 7.5 PH

Fentanyl 3.1 PH

Heroin – 5.3 PH

Cocaine – 6.3 PH

Toms Natural Toothpaste – 8.9 PH

Average Toothpaste – 5.5 PH

Death – 4.4 PH

Mass Murderers – 4.9 PH

Wine – 6.9 PH

Beer – 6.9 PH

Hard alcohol – 6.6 PH

Dr. Pepper – 76 PH

Diet Dr. Pepper – 6.5 PH

IBC root beer – 7.6 PH

Dad's root beer – 7.1 PH

Ginger ale – 7.5 PH

Coke – 7.1 PH diet – 6.4 PH

Big Red 6.9 PH

Mountain Dew – 5.4 diet 5.8PH

Pepsi – 5.9 PH diet – 6.8 PH

Nitroglycerine 2.1 PH

Kraft macaroni and cheese	4.3
GMO food	3.5
Arsenic	3.5
Cyanide	3.5
Tylenol	3.5 - Average cold 6.3
Nityl	4.1
Advil	6.4
Aspirin	7.1
Paint thinner	3.5
Paint	7.1 with lead 6.5
Antifreeze	3.5
Average Racists	6.3
Breast cancer	5.6 - Mammogram 5.1 Infrared Thermogram Infrared 9.1
Death	4.5
Transgender	5.1
Cancer death	5.3 - Average St. Jude patient 5.8
Miscarriage	5.3
Birth defects	5.8
Average F students	6.6
Average A students	9.2

Average Murderers	5.0 - Average mental patient 5.4
Average Illegal alien	6.3
Average Legal alien	8.5
Average Medicare/Medicaid	5.7
Average DUI or traffic accident	6.1
Average Divorce – 1 spouse	5.5
Gays (at birth)	6.3
Autism (at birth)	6.5
Down syndrome (at birth)	5.8
Automatic Death	4.4
Average Muslim	6.6
Average Jew	7.9
Average Mormon	8.1
Average Baptist	7.9
Average Hindu	7.5
Average Catholic	7.7
Average Methodist	8.3
Average farmers	9.1 It's easier to alkaline in the country
Average CNN reporter	5.5
Average Fox reporter	7.5
Sean Hannity	9.0

9.8 PH

Bed sheets with silver inlayed Silvadore sheets

Age 5 to death – gives energy and heals gall bladder, liver, pancreas, small intestines, lungs, glands, appendix, hearing, smell

If used in hospitals it will increase healing by 20%. Mattresses need to be changed more. If not, use mattress toppers.

The absence of gall bladder or tonsils makes the liver work 20% harder. Eat liver food with a minimum PH of 9. Increase the dosage by 20%.

When the appendix is removed eat stomach food with a minimum PH of 90. Increase the dosage by 30%.

Insulin users – eat pancreas food with a minimum PH of 9.2. Increase the dosage by 10%.

All disease is acidic with PH below 7
Alkaline PH 8 – 9.8 foods heal

Earth – Beef, bison, deer, lobster, oysters, mussels, scallops, fowl, goat, lamb
Capricorn, Taurus, Virgo

Air – Beef, bison, deer, flounder, Atlantic char, cod, grouper, halibut, 13 kinds of bass, goat, crab, shrimp, fowl

Aquarius, Gemini, Libra

Water – Flounder, Atlantic char, grouper, halibut, 13 kinds of bass, shrimp, cod, crab, fowl, pork, lamb, corn beef

Pisces, Cancer, Scorpio

Fire – Fowl, pork, lamb, beef, bison, deer, goat, lobster, oysters, scallops, mussels, corn beef

Aries, Leo, Sagittarius

If born on the cusp one day before or after sign changes, you can have both signs.

Only eat beef and pork raised and processed in the US. Avoid all food from China.

Burger King beef only 4.1 PH
Bojangles all meats 4.1 PH

Hardees all meats 4.3 PH
Taco Bell all meats 4.9 PH
DQ all meats 4.9 PH

9.0 PH

Apples – a neutral food (combine with all foods) – great for gall bladder, liver, nerves

Ages 5-25 1/3 day
Red Delicious – headache, PMS 1/day
4 days before period, skip 3 days then 1/day for 2 days
Granny apple – hiccups

Apple Juice – to stop swelling, as preventive medicine, drink 6oz before event/6oz after injury

9.5 PH

Artichoke – Pancreas, stomach, appendix, nerves, IQ, tonsils, blood, hearing, speech, sight,

Age 15 on - 5 ounces/3 days

9.0 PH

Asparagus – bones, lungs, stomach, gall bladder

Ages 8-25 5/5 days
Canned asparagus is ok.

9.5 PH

Bananas – Gall bladder, liver, lungs, bones, tonsils, appendix, teeth, sight, skin, spleen

Women – age 8 on 6 oz./2 days
Men – age 5 – 13 8 oz./2 days

At age 13 PH turns to 6.6

Pregnancy – 4 months 6 oz./2 days

For babies – gall bladder, stomach, tonsils, small intestine, glands, nerves, spleen, and brain

9.8 PH – the maximum PH

Beets – Liver, skin, taste, voice, pancreas, appendix, gall bladder

Age 5-25 5 ounces/3 day Makes great singers like Elvis – promotes constructive energy

9.5 PH

Bell Pepper – green, raw – bones, gall bladder, liver, pancreas, blood, lungs, heart, bones, teeth, small intestines, spleen

Age 5 – 25 5 oz./5 days

9.5 PH

Black Seed Oil – gall bladder, stomach, glands, teeth, blood, hearing

It kills parasites. It's great for removing addictions. 6 drops at bedtime with 4 oz. water for a maximum of 18 weeks. This works only with Amazing Herb brand in Buford, GA. It is the only one processed the right way.

Note: Because kidneys will fill up with waste take 2 milk thistles with black seed oil and then continue 12 days after you stop taking black seed oil to flush out the kidneys.

There are 43 kinds of parasites that know how to control the brain and can put you in pain if they don't get what they want. It's not you that is hooked on drugs, alcohol, sugar, etc. Get rid of the parasites and that will get rid of the cravings.

People who have the highest tolerance usually have the most parasites. There are people that can drive better with alcohol because the alcohol is giving the parasite their fix. They are not drunk because the parasites are absorbing the alcohol, but they won't pass a breathalyzer.

The breathalyzer is wrong over 50% of the time. But the lawyers make money. How about a law that anyone over 18 killing anyone with a motorized vehicle, drunk or not drunk, never operates a motorized vehicle again gets the death penalty. 30% drunk drivers kill again. 10% drunk drivers kill a 3rd time. That's why the mothers are MADD.

9.5 PH

Blueberries – gall bladder, liver, pancreas, bones, teeth, appendix, nerves, stomach, blood, nerves, smell, speech, brain, broken heart

Age 7 – 25 4 oz./3 days

Pregnancy – 6 oz./3 days

For babies – gall bladder, liver, pancreas, lungs, heart, bones, skin, blood, hair, nerves, IQ, smell, intestines.

9.5 PH

Broccoli – Gall bladder, brain, smell, lungs

Age 8 – 19 4 ounces/3 days
Age 25 on – for sleep 4 oz. at bedtime/4 weeks

9.5 PH

Brussel Sprouts – Skin, stomach, extra energy, gall bladder, glands, appendix, hearing, sight, speech

Age 8-25 5 sprouts/3 days
Extra energy 6 sprouts/day for up to 5 weeks

9.5 PH

Cantaloupe – Gall bladder, small intestines, nerves, heart, blood, glands, liver, teeth, appendix, brain

Age 21 – 5 ounces/3 days

9.5 PH

Cabbage – Gall bladder, small intestines, brain, hearing, blood, bones

Age 8 – 25 5 ounces/2 days

9.3 PH

Canola oil – gallbladder, eyes, glands, small intestine

Only alkaline frying oil

ACL, Achilles, and tendon tears are from too much fried food. Fry in alkaline canola oil.

9.5 PH

Carrots – Do not eat with peas - Brain, stomach, gall bladder

Age 8 -25 8 ounces/2 days eat raw or cook whole or 6" sections
Broken bones – 7 ounces/day without meat up to 45 days

9.8 PH Maximum PH

Castor Oil – your whole body – gall bladder, stomach, glands, skin, hair

Internal dose - age 5 – 25 1 tablespoon/5 days
Infectious diseases - 5 tablespoons/day for up to 9 days

External – each skin cell is 90% oxygen. If damaged cell has a minimum of 43% oxygen. You can restore the cell to 75% oxygen by rubbing castor oil into damaged area for 6 minutes. There will be a 6 hour chemical reaction replacing the oxygen. It may take up to 6 applications to reach 75%. It's great for anti-aging and 27 kinds of skin diseases. Birthmarks and tattoo removal can take up to 96 applications.

Hearing – put 12 drops in ear, let soak in for 15 minutes. Wait 6 hours. It may take up to 11 applications. See peanut oil.

Pregnancy – 6 months to weaned - 1 tablespoon/day

For babies – gall bladder, liver, pancreas, small intestines, heart, glands, teeth

9.5 PH

Cauliflower – brain food – teeth, gallbladder, liver, stomach, appendix, pancreas, pollen - ages 5 – 19 4 oz./day a must

Combat chemo – start 5 days before 1st treatment
Cauliflower – 5oz/day
Daikon - 5oz/day
Yellow squash – 5oz/day
Mango – 6oz/day
Green bell peppers (raw) – 1/day

9.4 PH

Cherries – pancreas, smell, small intestine, lungs, appendix, tonsils

Ages 8 to 25 – 20 cherries/3 days

Pregnancy - gallbladder, liver, pancreas, small intestine, appendix, speech, skin, kidneys

4 months to weaned – 10 cherries/2 days

For babies – gall bladder

8.9 PH

Coconut – Gall bladder, stomach, blood, tonsils, pancreas, appendix, IQ

Women – From age 5 on - 1 oz./3 days
Men – From age 6 on - 13 1 oz./2 days – at age 13 PH turns to 6.6

Pregnancy - 6 months to weaned - 1 oz./2 days

For babies - gall bladder, small intestines, heart, teeth, skin, hearing, blood, nerves

9.5 PH – Black

Coffee – Gall Bladder, stomach, teeth, voice, small intestines, ears, smelling, blood, eyes, liver

Age 8 on 6 oz./day

Using dairy with coffee upsets the digestive system. Use nondairy creamer. The best tenderizer for beef is ground up coffee. Cover on both sides and wait for a minimum of 3 hours. You'll be surprised.

The best fertilizer for plants is used coffee grounds.

Pregnancy – 5 month to weaned 6 oz./day

For babies – Pancreas, stomach, gall bladder, voice, spleen, liver, brain

9.5 PH

Corn – nerves, smell, gall bladder, glands, liver, pancreas, teeth, heart, stomach, appendix, tonsils, eyes

Age 4 – 15 5 oz./3days best if cooked in shuck

9.5 PH

Daikon – hair, bones, tonsils, glands, eyes, gallbladder, small intestine, lungs

Ages 6-21 4oz/week
Chemo – 5oz/day – start 5 days before treatment
Balding – 4oz/week
Broken bones – 10oz/3 days – avoid all meat, meat suppresses healing eat 1 lemon/day

Pregnancy – starting at month 5 until weaned – 4oz/3 days

For babies – brain, IQ and smell
Eyes, ears, small intestine, teeth, lungs, skin, voice

8.9 PH

Liquid Echinacea – smell, stomach, glands age 9 – 21 2 drops/day

Sore throat - 5 drops. Capsules don't work. It has to be liquid or you could eat the plant.

9.8 PH Maximum PH

Eggs – pancreas, small intestines, blood, teeth, appendix, nerves, tonsils, hearing, liver, skin

Age 8 on 2/day
Eat the whole egg. It is 35 times harder to digest an egg yolk without the whites. Undigested food turns to fat.

9.5 PH

Figs – Pancreas, stomach, tonsils, speech

Ages 5 – 25 5 ounces/2 days

Pregnancy – 5 months to weaned 5 ounces/5 days

For babies teeth, speech, eyes, nerves, tonsils, voice

9.1 PH if prepared right

Garlic – Gall Bladder, stomach, teeth, colon, bones, skin, hair, nerves, spleen, voice

Age 6-21 1 clove/4 days
Crush clove. Let air hit it for 10 minutes, then use within 30 minutes

Pregnancy – 8 months to weaned – 1 clove/day

For babies, pancreas, stomach, liver, heart, bones, glands, hair, brain

9.8 PH maximum PH

Ginseng – brain, pancreas, bones, nerves, lungs, gall bladder, stomach, smell, eyes, ears

Age 8 – 20 3 capsules/2 days with 4 oz. water

9.5 PH

Gluten – to function proper your pancreas and stomach needs gluten.

There are 3 kinds of parasites (invented in 1993) that disrupt the gluten intake. To remove them take 4 drops of black seed oil from Amazing Herbs in 4 oz. of water at bedtime for 10 days. To flush out the waste in the kidneys take 2 milk thistles for 20 days.

Pancreas and stomach function 20% better with gluten adding 5 years to your lifespan with 20% more joy. The body needs gluten.

9.5 PH

Greens (Spinach) – Gall bladder, small intestines, heart, teeth, lungs

Age 5 – 25 5 ounces/3 days

Pregnancy 6 months to weaned – 8 ounces/2 days

For babies – brain, higher IQ, smell, lungs

9.5 PH

Beans – liver, IQ, pancreas, stomach, gallbladder

Green beans – circulation and sex drive

Pinto, navy, baked, azuki, legumes, lentils (all beans)
Age 9 on – 4oz/2 days

9.0 PH

Green Grapes – Gall Bladder, stomach, heart, bones, teeth, glands, hearing, sight, voice

Age 3 – 21 5 grapes/days
To reduce EMF poison or radiation poison - 15 grapes/day for up to 3 months

Green Olives – Gall bladder, eyes, liver, skin

Age 12 – 25 5/2 day

Pregnancy – 8 months to weaned – 5/day

For babies – gall bladder, eyes, small intestine, glands, teeth, blood, nerves, skin, heart

9.6 PH

Green peas – do not eat with carrots – gallbladder, liver, voice, teeth, appendix, tonsils, blood, nerves, IQ, ears, builds muscles. A must

Ages 5-25 – 10 peas/day or 25/3 days

Pregnancy – 5th months to weaned – 30 peas/3 days

For babies – pancreas, gallbladder, small intestine, IQ, liver

9.3 PH

Hawthorne Berries – teeth, gall bladder, liver, glands, sight

Age 45 on – 1/week
Toothache – 3/day up to 4 months
25% of all diseases start with tooth decay

8.5 PH

Hazelnut with Marion berry only from Oregon because of the Oregon soil – gall bladder, liver, pancreas, eyes, smell

American Indians have parasites in their sperm and eggs. These parasites are allergic to alcohol which is why they did not sell fire water to the Indians. To get rid of these parasites and hold your liquor take 4/day for 55 days for females – 5/day for 75 days for males

"Hay Ya Ya Ya Ya Ya Ya Ya Ya
Hay Ya Ya Ya Ya Ya Ya Ya"

9.8 PH maximum PH

Holy Basil – gall bladder, liver, stomach, brain, heart, bones, glands, nerves, hearing

Age 8 – 25 3 capsules/2 days with 4 oz. water

9.5 PH - After 3 days raw is 9.0 PH

Honey – Gall bladder, liver, taste, hearing, shin, hair, lungs, reduces anger

Age 10 – 19 2 tablespoons/3 days

9.5 PH

Honeydew Melons – Pancreas, stomach, hearing, smell, liver, small intestines

Age 5 – 21 5 ounces/3 days

8.9 PH

Lavender oil – pancreas, worry, fear

Age 8 on – 5 drops/3days in 4 oz. water

Pregnancy – 8 month to weaned 2 drops/day 4 oz. water

For babies liver, pancreas, tonsils

Lemons – gall bladder, stomach, nerves, teeth, ears, small intestine

Age 5 on - 1/2 day
Healing bones – 1/day maximum 50 days
2 lemons with no more than 7 oz. of water to a meal with pineapple adds 1 alkaline.
You can use 7 oz. of Simply Lemonade.

Pregnancy – 4 months to weaned – 1/day
For babies – gall bladder, stomach, nerves, teeth, ears, small intestine, glands

9.8 PH

Mango – Nitrogen, liver, smell, ears, eyes

68% blacks – Ages 11 – 18 4oz./day, ages 18 – 25 11 oz./day, ages 25 on 15 oz./day

Sickle cell is lack of nitrogen. The air in Africa is 15% nitrogen, in Cuba it's 13%.

Without nitrogen the body starts deteriorating the brain. 98% of the black people in jail are nitrogen deficient. All black people at age 33 – 35 should take a vacation in Africa (the best is south central Africa) for 2 weeks minimum. If it's too expensive, go to Cuba and go barefoot or wear open sandals for the maximum effect. The average black persons PH that goes to jail is 6.3 and 6.1 PH when they get out. They go in angry and come out angrier creating more repeated customers. There is no excuse for anyone released from jail not to have a PH of 8.3.

56% Hispanic, American Indian, Eskimo

Ages 5 – 12 2 oz./day, ages 12 – 25 4 oz./day, ages 25 – death 6 oz./day
These people need air to be 5% nitrogen and 5% sulfur.

For 68% blacks its age is 32. For 68% Hispanics its age is 36. Depending on race with the proper nitrogen or nitrogen/Sulphur combination making the right air then raise the age to 44. People who leave their birth countries unless representing their birth country are really never joyful and resent us, especially if they are takers instead of givers. With the air south of the Rio Grande River, mangos supply the nitrogen. Sulfur comes from fowl because it takes sulfur to make feathers. It is healthier and a more joyful life to breathe the right air. Without it you will start aging faster at age 32. Alaska air is 8% sulfur so Eskimos only need nitrogen provided by salmon. The US should stop illegal aliens for coming over the border for their own health or send them to Alaska. You could say don't forget to remember the Alamo or you'll be rubbing noses with the Eskimos. To be an asset to America, people applying for citizenship should have a PH of a minimum 8.5.

Motorcycle deaths are less than 1/100 of 1% of the traffic but 9% of the deaths. 8% is after the 44th birthday for whites, 33rd for blacks and 36th for Hispanics. Those that don't have any problems started riding before the age of 21.

Maple syrup grade B 8.8 PH grade A 8.6 PH

Pancreas, stomach, glands, tonsils, appendix, blood, eyes, smell, liver

Ages 8 to 23 – 4 tablespoons/2 days
Pregnancy at 8 months - pancreas, stomach, teeth, appendix, skin, bone, heart, spleen, voice

9.5 PH

Milk Thistle – small intestine, kidneys, liver, spleen, pancreas, stomach, bones, teeth, skin, hair, nerves

Age 6 on - 1 capsule/4 days

If there is a puffiness or darkness under the eyes you need to clean out the kidneys. 5/days with 4 oz. water for up to 6 days

9.8 PH

Mineral Oil – skin, gall bladder, small intestines, stomach, brain, bone, heart, teeth, tonsils, smell, appendix, blood, aura

Diarrhea 4 tablespoons – Must be at least 10 years old and weigh at least 80 pounds

Age 45 – 65 1 tablespoon/3 days at bedtime
Age 65 – 75 2 tablespoons/3 days at bedtime
Age 75 – death 2 tablespoons/2 days at bedtime

People with soul groups have 1,000 strands of aura. 200 strands go to 5 separate sets of organs. 30 strands go from heart to pancreas to brain. When 25 strands break you die from Alzheimer's. Take 3 tablespoons at bedtime for 10 days then skip 4 days. 70 strands gall bladder to liver up to 10 weeks. 50 strands small to large intestines up to 4 weeks. 30 strands large intestine to lungs 10 applications up to 8 weeks. It may take up to 18 weeks.

9.3 PH

Mushrooms – Gall bladder, small intestines, heart, liver, stomach, appendix, tonsils, nerves,

Age 5 on 3 oz./4 days

8.3 PH

Nuts – teeth, blood, pancreas, small intestines, gallbladder

Meats for vegans –no more than 4oz/day
Age 12 on – 4oz/day

9.5 PH

Okra – nerves, pancreas, smell, eyes, voice, liver, teeth, brain

Ages 5-25 1/day or 3/3 days
Add up to 8" in height
Only fry with canola oil 9.3 PH

9.8 PH maximum PH

Olive Oil – spleen, brain, gall bladder, liver, stomach, bone, teeth, glands, skin

Age 4 on 1 tablespoon/day
Note: Do not heat. When heated the PH changes to 6.6.

9.5 PH

Onions – gall bladder, voice, liver, pancreas, heart, bones, teeth, glands, small intestines, smell

Age 6 – 39 5 oz./3 days

9.5 PH

Oranges – Liver, lungs, gall bladder, glands, teeth, appendix, blood

Age 5 – 25 3 ounces/day
From age 35 on 5 ounces/day for stomach

Pregnancy – 8 months to weaned 5 ounces/day

For babies gall bladder, stomach, heart, bones, liver, pancreas, lungs, glands, tonsils, appendix, blood, IQ, hearing, nerves, skin

9.1 PH

Peaches – A neutral food that combines with all foods. Blood pressure, blood clots, gall bladder, pancreas, stomach, teeth, colds

From age 5 on 5/week canned is ok

Pregnancy – 5 month to weaned 1/day

For babies – Pancreas, stomach, spleen, tonsils, heart, blood, nerves, skin, heart, voice, liver, small intestines

9.5 PH

Peanut Oil – pancreas, stomach, tonsils,

Internal age 45 – 65 1 tablespoon/5 days

External – each skin cell is 90% oxygen. If the damaged cell is below 43% oxygen you can restore the cell to 70% oxygen by rubbing peanut oil into the damaged area for 4 minutes. There will be a 6 hour chemical reaction restoring the oxygen into the cell. It may take up to 12 applications, then 2 applications of castor oil to go to 75%.

See castor oil.

Football Concussions – on the left side starting 1" before the temple to back, 8" to 9" starting at the hair line at the ear go up 5". It may take up to 7 applications and 3 castor oil applications. Use the helmet with 8 3/4" holes and add 1/2 padding, especially on the left side of the brain which mostly effects the liver, but also the pancreas, small intestines, lungs, stomach. See apple juice.

Ruptured ear drum – put 5 drops in ear, let absorb for 10 minutes. Wait 6 hours and repeat. It will take between 5 – 8 applications. Then put 12 drops of castor oil. Let soak in for 15 minutes, wait 6 hours. It will take 4 applications.

C-section – open wounds – 15 applications of peanut oil and 8 of castor oil.

9.0 PH

Pears – Skin, nerves, being upset, gall bladder, liver, heart, teeth, appendix, speech

Age 5 on 1/day
If having a really bad day, 2 canned pears are ok.

8.9 PH

Pepper – gallbladder, bones, teeth, glands, lungs

Age 5 on – 2 teaspoons/day

9.5 PH

Pineapple – Pancreas, increases meat by .5 alkaline, it can make an acidic meal alkaline, glands, stomach, eyes, IQ, brain

Age 8 on - 3 oz./meal adds .5 alkaline – with 2 lemons add 1 alkaline

9.7 PH

Plums – Gall bladder, skin, stomach, glands, teeth, appendix, tonsils, hair, voice, taste

Age 4 on – 1/3 day
For memory – 2 plums/day for 12 days

Pregnancy – 3 months to weaned 1/day until weaned

For babies – gall bladder, stomach, pancreas, liver, small intestines

9.0 PH

Potatoes – Gall Bladder, colon, stomach, heart

Age 7 on 6 ounces/3 days

9.8 PH

Quinoa – the only high alkaline grain – gall bladder, blood, IQ

Age 5 to 25 4 oz., 5 days

9.5 PH

Raspberries – Glands, pancreas, gall bladder, stomach, taste, smells

Age 8 – 25 4 berries/5 days

Pregnancy – 8 berries per day, 5th month to babies birth holds womb up, prevents stretch marks

For babies – gall bladder, blood, heart, voice

9.3 PH

Salt – gall bladder, small intestine, bones, teeth, tonsils, nerves

Age 11 on – 1 teaspoon/day

O blood – table salt is best. For all other blood types, sea salt is best. If not, change PH to 8.6.

9.3 PH

Soy Milk – gall bladder, smell, intestines, heart, glands, tonsils, blood, hair, eyes, skin, hearing, liver

Age 4 – 20 3 oz./day

Do not take chocolate with soy. It is 5 times harder to digest.

To make breast bigger, from age 12 years, 6 months to 13 years, 6 months 3 oz./day. No more or you will need a breast reduction. Athletes need to avoid soy milk.

9.5 PH

Squash – pancreas, bones, skin, blood, hair, brain

Age 12 – 25 4 oz./2 days

Pregnancy – 3 months to weaned 6 oz./2 days

For babies – gall bladder, liver, pancreas, stomach, glands, blood, smell, eyes, ears, brain

9.6 PH

Sweet Potatoes – Pancreas, smell, spleen, small intestines, gall bladder, IQ, hearing, eyes, speech

Age 12 – death 10 oz./4 days
Note: Avoid cinnamon if you have a fungus (like nail fungus)

Pregnancy – 8 months to weaned 10 oz./4 days with a tablespoon of cinnamon

For babies – Pancreas, stomach, teeth, speech, ears, eyes, IQ, nerves

9.5PH

Tapioca – gall bladder, liver, pancreas, glands, tonsils, colitis

Age 12 on – 1 oz./2 days

Pregnancy – 8 months to weaned 2/day

For babies – gall bladder, liver, pancreas, teeth, smell, small intestines

9.6 PH

Thyme – gallbladder, small intestine, lungs, teeth, smell, brain

Age 5 on – 1 capsule/day with 4oz water or ¼ oz. in food per day

9.5 PH

Tomatoes – gall bladder, liver, pancreas, worry

Age 8 on 3 oz. every 4 days

9.5 PH

Turmeric – pancreas, bones, teeth, nerves, kidney, blood, smell

Ages 8 – 25 3 capsules/5 days

Pregnancy – 5 months to weaned 3 capsules/3 days

For babies – gall bladder, liver, pancreas, stomach, nerves, smell, eyes ears, brain

7.7 PH

Cigarettes – American Spirit has no chemical – **Cigars** 6.9 PH

6.6 PH

Cigarettes with chemicals – Do you know the chemicals put in cigarettes are what are used to make LSD. Change to an alkaline brand.

After major operations, to heal, stop smoking for 6 months. Cigarettes will stop the healing process.

7.5 PH

Marijuana – gall bladder, liver, lungs, glands, appendix, and hair

From age 45 on for 23% of the population it does not affect everyone.

From age 31 on it compensates for lack of nitrogen in the air.

For those it does affect, it opens up your crown chakra making you more spiritual.

9.5 PH

Dog Food – Ol'Roy – complete nutrition – age 2 on

Dog's/puppies need dry food without vegetables or fruit. If they need any vegetables they'll eat grass. The same is for cats.

Cat – Short hair cats need wet food. Long hair cats need dry food.

Note: You can have the best quality ingredients, but if not processed the right way, it can turn alkaline into acidic.

The only alkaline dogs

Collie (Lassie) 7.7 PH Akita 8.1 PH Japanese Akita 8.3 PH St. Bernard 8.6 PH with alcohol 8.5 PH, Cats – Acidic – 6.8 PH

9.8 PH maximum PH

Breast milk – gall bladder, liver, pancreas, brain, nerves, bones, teeth, glands, tonsils, stomach, heart, skin, hair, spleen

8 to 13 oz./day – best 3 feeds a day for 8 months if sore apply up to 5 applications of castor oil. See castor oil. Women with a PH of at least 8.5 should not have any problem breast feeding. If not, use no more than 4 oz. of formula a day. Follow with Carnation milk.

Confucius said that the end depends on the beginning. Babies need breast feeding mentally and physically. Their IQ is 20% higher. 4 out of 5 prisoners were not breast fed. Now less than half of the babies are breast fed. When prayer was in schools 95% of the babies were breast fed. Males that are not breast fed are the ones that are obsessed with breasts as an adult.

9.8 PH maximum PH

Carnation Condensed Milk – Breast fed babies are easier to be alkaline and stay alkaline and balanced throughout life. Carnation condensed milk is the closest milk to breast milk equal to 88%. If not breastfed give baby 4 oz. of formula per day followed by carnation milk for the first 7 months, then 3 months of carnation milk and then weaned. Cow's milk is 8.3 PH with 20% human breast milk. Goat milk is 8.8 PH with 35%. Mothers who breast feed need to have a PH of at least 8.3. The baby needs to be held 8 hours a day total by the mother or female blood relatives and the father 30 minutes a day or male blood relatives for the first 10 months. There should be zero alcohol intake from month 2 of pregnancy to weaned.

Breast Cancer is usually caused from metal buildup in the left kidney, probably from iron by eating too much meat. Take 3 raw green peppers for breakfast for 55 days with 2 milk thistle for 73 days. Breast feeding reduces chance of cancer by 35%. Breast implants - 9.5 PH gall bladder food increasing the dosage by 20%.

Rubber Soul by The Beatles

aura, brain, lungs,

Pregnancy 7 months – 1/day until born

For babies – spirituality increases 35%

The Power of the Cook

The enzymes of the cook go into the food. After a year you are addicted to these enzymes. This is why you crave your mother's cooking. If the cooks PH is below 7.5 it will be just the opposite. One of the main reasons separations do not work is because of food withdrawals.

9.59 PH

Charcoal tablets – kills all bacteria, great for food poisoning, must replace good bacteria. 5 oz. kefir (not strawberry or peach) – 5.9 PH

Other 9.1 PH is blueberry, blackberry, pomegranate

Burns

Peanut oil up to 5 applications
Castor oil up to 5 applications

Light bulbs

Mercury light bulbs 4.5 PH
Regular light bulbs 9.5 PH
GE Shelby light bulbs 9.7 PH last a hundred years

EMF is from mercury light bulbs. They cause damage to babies' gall bladder, liver, heart, teeth and bones. This is especially true for babies under 25 pounds.

Anti-EMF food is plums 8-9 PH, 1 oz. of plum juice for 5 days for babies over 10 pounds. Some symptoms are ears stick out; they sleep less than 8 hours a day. For the first 10 months babies should sleep 12 hours a day.

The easiest way to test your alkaline PH is with PH balance strips.

Other Books by the Author:

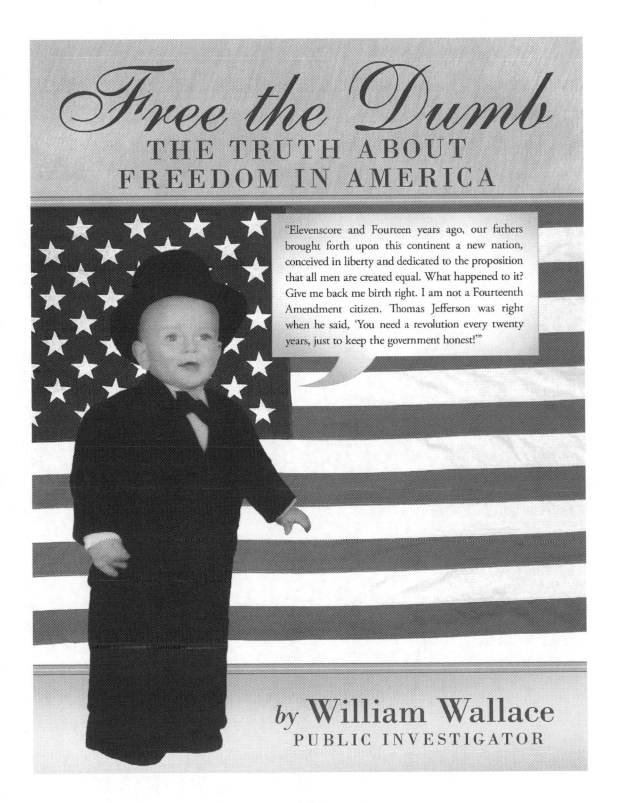

Free the Dumb

Printed in the United States
By Bookmasters